Weight Reduction
& much more!

Weight Reduction & much more!

WITH THETA HEALING

Lorraine Knight

To order additional copies of this book, contact:
Xlibris Corporation
0-800-644-6988
www.xlibrispublishing.co.uk
Orders@xlibrispublishing.co.uk
302521

CONTENTS

FOREWORD

Why had my weight, size and shape become such an issue and a focus in my life?

I wanted to get off the constant thoughts about how I looked; food, calories and yo-yo dieting.

I wanted freedom.

I decided that, for me, I needed to find the answer to solve my own issues, looking at all the tools and techniques I could muster to finally becoming my ideal weight.

I also recognised the benefits of Theta healing, and how everyone can benefit even if you do not want to become a Theta Practitioner.

I had what you may call a 'normal life' but finally began a spiritual journey when, after surgery, I received a Reiki session to alleviate pain. I found the physical sensation of Reiki without physical contact fascinating and, following a spiritual awakening, I decided to study to become a Reiki Master. This was an inspirational spiritual journey which, in time, led me to discover and experience the powerful healing modality of Theta healing.

Having witnessed the awesome results that Theta can achieve, I studied in the UK and the Netherlands to become a Theta Practitioner and then to become a Theta Teacher.

It was during one of my sessions with a client that I realised that it was the subconscious beliefs that I held within me that were the cause of my never ending battles with dieting and I decided that Theta was the ideal tool to help end this "war with weight".

I began by creating a one day Theta healing workshop aimed at providing new tools and techniques to understand the reasons as to why people carry excess weight. These started in early 2010, and it was at one of these workshops that a client suggested that it would be a good idea to get the workshop out and available to as many people as possible, maybe on a CD or even in a book, so here it is!

There may be many factors that attribute to our size and shape, so this book has different sections covering many aspects such as clearing beliefs, healing from past traumas, creating new feelings and much, much more. Although primarily aimed at helping people to find, understand and change the subconscious beliefs that cause them to retain weight, the Theta techniques used go much deeper and can be used in all areas of people's lives. The journey that you are about to embark upon is one of discovery in more ways than just focusing on your weight. You will experience techniques that can be used to discover and let go of subconscious blocks that may be holding you back in many other areas of your life.

During this book I will refer to "Downloads" and "Macros".
A "Download" is used to describe the process of receiving all that has been asked for from Source Energy. This is very similar to when you download information from the internet to your computer.

When asking for a belief change from Source Energy, there are various components that we ask to be included in the process, e.g. "I have Source's perspective, definition and understanding of . . . ." or "I know when to, how to and it is possible to . . . .".

To simplify and include all components in the healing process, we pull them all together into a "Macro" such as "Teach it" or "Change this belief".

To get the most value out of this book, I would suggest that you only try using the techniques described after you have read the whole book.

WHAT IS THETA HEALING?

A full description of what Theta healing is and what it can do is worth a book in its own right and, indeed, there are several books on the market which will provide you with the A to Z of Theta healing, so this is just a brief overview.

Theta healing was founded in 1995 by Vianna Stibal who cured herself of Cancer.

It is based on the acceptance that there is a higher divine Consciousness in the Universe, often referred to as God, Source, Universal Energy or Creator of All That Is.

It is not based on any religion, but on an acceptance, or faith, that there is a higher Source Energy.

As Theta practitioners we ask 'Creator of All That Is' to carry out the healing, and our part is to witness it taking place. We are always connected to Source Energy, and it's our birthright, so each and every one of us can do this.

Before understanding how Theta works, we must first understand a bit more about our brains. There are 5 basic brain wave states, and these are described in the table below:

5 Brain wave states

Alpha	More relaxed, the bridge between Beta and Theta (brain waves 7—14 cycles per second)
Beta	Thinking and communicating (brain waves 14—28 cycles per second)

Delta	Deep sleep (brain waves slowed to 0-4 cycles per second)
Gamma	When we are processing information (from 40—5000 cycles per second)
Theta	A very deep state of relaxation, which is used in hypnosis (4-7 cycles per second)

To connect to the Creator of All That Is, we need to let go of our ego and, to be able to do this, we need to get out of "our space", this being achieved by going into the Theta Brain Wave State. Initially, we use a meditation to help us go into the Theta Brain Wave State but, with practice it becomes possible to connect in an instant.

It may sound a bit daunting to say that the role of a Theta Practitioner is to witness or see the healing take place, which is a vision in our mind's eye but, if we can imagine a walk to the shops, then we can imagine and witness the healing.

In the foreword you were able to read that Theta healing can be used to recognise and work with beliefs that are held in our subconscious. So, I hear you ask, if these beliefs and blocks are held in my subconscious, how can I recognise them in the first place?

Firstly, we need to understand that all of our beliefs are held on four distinct levels, and it may be necessary to heal on any or even all of these levels. The levels of belief are:

➢ Beliefs from this lifetime, which are our core beliefs
➢ Beliefs from past lifetimes e.g. I believe that there is a famine, which is one of the possibilities why I may store excess fat in my body
➢ Genetic beliefs that come through our DNA, having been passed down from our ancestors and
➢ Beliefs held on our soul level, which is all that we are.

Studies have shown that, when we state a truth that is held in our subconscious our muscles become stronger and, inversely, if we tell a lie or make a statement that our subconscious does not believe, then our muscles become weaker.

To be able to access our subconscious mind, we use an energy test which can be used to confirm the beliefs that we hold. This energy test works even if our conscious mind may disagree, and can be used to confirm that the healing has been completed.

This energy test is also used in Kinesiology and is known as the "Muscle Test". How this works is described in the next section.

MUSCLE TESTING

The Muscle Test is the window to our subconscious mind so to understand what is in there we need to get it right. There are two different types of Muscle Test that can be carried out, one when we are standing up, and one that involves using our hands. Both versions are equally valid, however some people find one or the other to be more effective. Try them both and use the one that is easier for you.

Before trying the Muscle Test, there are three things that you need to note:

> Being well hydrated brings better results, so ensure you are hydrated and drink plenty of water. If you still encounter any problems with the muscle test, then rub your kidneys.
> The subconscious mind has a problem with negatives and may give strange results, so avoid negative statements with " 't ", such as can't, don't, not, isn't, won't, shouldn't.
> When starting to muscle test, it helps if you are facing north.

You will use muscle testing throughout the book to see what negative subconscious beliefs you hold, what emotions you are still holding onto and to confirm that the healing has taken place

MUSCLE TEST—STANDING UP

This is how you muscle test when standing up:

> ➤ Stand upright, feet slightly apart, body relaxed
> ➤ Whilst standing perfectly balanced repeat the word 'yes, yes, yes' and allow your body to move. As your muscles strengthen your body should sway forward.
> ➤ Repeat this using the word 'no, no, no', and your body should sway backwards as the muscles weaken.
> ➤ Test with statements that are both true and false, like 'I live in . . . .' 'I am wearing . . . .' 'My name is . . . .'
> ➤ Make sure you have this working before you go on

MUSCLE TEST—USING HANDS

This is how you muscle test by using your hands:

> ➤ If you are right-handed, place your left hand palm up. Now connect the tip of your left thumb with the tip of your left index finger. If you are left-handed, place your right hand palm up. Now connect the tip of your right thumb with the tip of your right index finger. These are often called the "Circuit Fingers".
> ➤ Now place the thumb and index finger of the other hand inside the 'loop' that you created in the above step. These should be right under your 'looped' thumb and index finger, just touching them. These are often called the "Test Fingers".
> ➤ Keeping this position, apply even pressure on the Circuit Fingers and, while repeating the word 'yes', try and prise open the 'Loop' with your Test Fingers. Then repeat this

exercise using the word 'no' and see if you can feel a
difference in pressure or strength between the two
words.

➢ Correct muscle testing would be that for 'yes' the Circuit
Fingers will be strong and be harder to prise open and, for
'no', the Circuit Fingers will be weak and be easier to prise
open..

HOW TO USE THIS BOOK TO DO YOUR OWN HEALING DOWNLOADS.

Using a 'Download' in Theta healing is very similar to using a download to your computer from the Internet. On the Internet you ask for information to be downloaded to your computer from its source. In Theta healing we ask for the healing to be 'downloaded' from the Source Energy to us.

As with the Internet, there are certain steps that need to be taken to ensure that Theta healing downloads are received and stored properly and, in this section, I will walk you through the steps you need to take to use this book to begin healing yourself and changing your own beliefs. These steps are not just limited to the subject covered by this book, but can be used for any other healings you may wish to ask for.

1. The first thing to note is to remember that Theta healing is not linked to any religion, but does rely on a belief that there is a Source Energy. Whatever or whoever you believe in, and however you refer to this needs to replace my words of 'Creator of All That Is' or 'God'

2. To do your own healings you will need to practice connecting to the 'Creator of All That Is'. Until you have become proficient in this connection, it is best to use the meditations provided and you can do this in various ways.
   a. Have someone you know and trust to read the meditation to you.
   b. Record your own voice and replay it to yourself
   c. You may wish to purchase the accompanying CD that has all the Meditations available on it.

3. When you are ready to start the downloads remember to test each belief individually stating them out aloud and using the muscle test technique you chose previously, e.g.

   I have the overweight gene = (Yes or No)

4. Looking at the 'How to set a Macro' section at the end of the book, it is a good idea to decide what you are asking to receive from 'Creator of All That Is' with all the healings you do. You will only need to decide this once as, after that, you can use the macro to cover all the components.

5. To make it easy, before you are ready to connect to 'Creator of All That Is', read out the command as it is stated in the book and a list of beliefs you wish to change. Then, when you go to 'Creator of All That Is' just state *"as I have just read out for my highest and best good, and in the highest and best way, thank you, it is done, it is done, it is done. Show me"*.

6. Before you try and receive downloads, I would suggest that you read the whole book. However, you may need to go over the book a few times to get all the healing downloads. The main reason for this is that our subconscious beliefs are like building blocks, the more we heal, the more the blocks are removed, and the more the likelihood that we uncover additional blocks that need to be addressed. Therefore, some sections that appear later on in the book may help with any of the early beliefs that did not change. Please note that, if a belief didn't change first time around, there is a good chance that you have a stronger, deeper seated belief or issue holding it in place.

7. Once you have made the command to have the healing, allow in your mind's eye, your imagination to see what ever you see. We all have the right to co-create with 'Source

Energy' so we are all are able do it. Our job is to be the witness to the healing in anyway that happens for us, and to help us achieve this, we have Clairaudience, Clairvoyance, Clairsentience, and Claircognizance. Therefore, no matter what we use to witness—from colours, lights, full blown movies, a feeling, a knowing, or just a flash in the pan, just witness the occurrence with no doubts. As often stated in a well known advert for sports equipment, Just Do It! Allow 'Creator of All That Is' to do the healings and allow you to be the witness. Don't forget to leave enough time to witness the healing through to completion—you'll just know when it's done.

8. Always remember that you can always ask 'Creator of All That Is' for anything at anytime.

9. If a healing didn't happen, remember there are probably stronger, deep seated subconscious beliefs that are holding it in place. We will learn more about this as we go through the book.

10. If you fear letting go or are unsure of any healing then ask 'Creator of All That Is' what would happen if you did allow yourself to heal from this now or know this now? This is a good way to clear some of those deeper seated blocks.

11. As you become more proficient at connecting to 'Creator of All That Is' it can become as quick as you wish it to be. So go at your own speed and once your subconscious mind knows the process to connect and how easy it is to connect to 'Creator of All That Is', you may just need to say the word 'God' or whatever works for you, and you'll be there.

12. This book is made up of many exercises to heal and discover what is it for you that prevents you reducing your weight, but also, I have added many additional negative and

positive beliefs that will help with the journey to becoming your ideal weight in the section 'Other downloads you may wish to check'

13. Connecting to the 'Creator of All That Is' is a journey through the seven planes of existence. The journey is a bit like travelling through the veils of each plane. You can find out more about the seven planes in various books and the internet but, basically, they are:

1st	Crystals and Minerals
2nd	Plants
3rd	Humans
4th	Spirits
5th	Ascended masters; Jesus, Buddha, Reiki Masters
6th	The Laws
7th	Creator of all that is

MEDITATION TO 'CREATOR OF ALL THAT IS'

This meditation has been designed to help you connect to 'Creator of All That Is'. You will be able to use this meditation for all your healings as you go forward, however once proficient at connecting to source energy you will be able to connect in an instant.

If you are able to relax and visualise easily you can begin at **Journey to the Seventh Plane** below without doing the initial part of the meditation.

Close your eyes and begin to relax . . . take a deep breath in . . . . allow yourself to just focus on your breath . . . . Breathing deep and slow . . . deep and slow . . . allow yourself to relax more and more . . . .

And now just take your awareness to your body . . . allowing your body to relax as every muscle in your body begins to soften and relax . . . . .

Sink down into the chair . . . and relax more . . . now starting with your head . . . . just allow all the muscles in your head and face to relax . . . just soothing and relaxing . . . more relaxed than before

And the muscles in your shoulders and arms begin to relax . . . . relaxing more . . . . and more . . . allowing the relaxation to seep over your body . . . .

And with each breath you take . . . . you relax more and more . . . now further down . . . through to your arms and even further . . . . all the way down to the tips of your fingers . . . .

Allowing that relaxation to bring a sense of calm and peace . . . . . and now the muscles in your chest and back begin to fully relax . . . as you breath deeper and deeper . . . . .
And more of your body just settles . . . settles into a more relaxed state than before . . . . and even your breathing just relaxes . . . more and more you just relax, as feelings of comfort begin to surround you . . . .

As you drift into a more relaxed state than before . . . . .you allow yourself just to focus on my voice . . . . as you relax more . . . .

And now your legs, all the way down past your shins . . . into your feet . . . and down to the tips of your toes your body relaxes . . . .
.

And you drift deeper and deeper, relaxing more and more with every breath you take . . . just drift deeper and deeper . . . .

Deeper and deeper . . . .

Journey to Seventh Plane

Now I want you to imagine . . . . imagine that your feet are firmly on the floor . . . firmly grounding you to the floor . . . and allow your imagination to drift as your awareness goes even further down . . . connecting . . . .

Connecting to the earth . . . further down . . . all the way passing through to the roots of the trees . . . further down and relaxing more with every breath you take . . .

You imagine yourself going further still . . . while safe in this space . . . . your awareness goes even further . . . . and you relax even more . . . .

And as you go further, you see this beautiful crystal in the middle of the earth . . . you can touch this beautiful crystal with your feet . . . grounding you safely to the earth . . . .

And now, still connected safely to the earth, your awareness comes back up through your body . . . up through your legs . . . relaxing your muscles even more . . . . so that if there were still tensions in your body . . . . they are now gone . . . moving up through your feet . . . .

Up your legs . . . through all your muscles . . . relaxing more . . . releasing more . . . as the energy comes up your body . . . .

It strengthens . . . more energy . . . moving up . . . . your awareness now rises up through your body . . . . More and more energy gathers . . . and all your energy centres, chakras are opened and cleansed . . . . coming up higher through your body relaxing you more and more . . . as your energy gathers your awareness comes up to the top of your head . . . .

And you find yourself in your own beautiful bubble of light . . . protected and safe . . . you may notice the colours in that beautiful bubble . . . . .

And in your bubble of light you go up . . . up and up . . . past the stars and planets . . . and up even further . . . through layers and layers . . . .

Through dark light . . . and light . . . . through dark light . . . and light . . . you may see ancestors . . . you may even ask them to help you . . . . or you may just go past . . . .

Up closer and closer . . . further and further . . . and then you see a brighter light and here you enter a thicker jelly like substance . . . which is where all the laws of the universe are held . . . and your bubble bursts . . . you are safe . . . and free . . . and you find yourself swimming or moving further up . . . . up and up . . .

And then you see this beautiful iridescent white light. .and you go closer and closer through the entrance . . . and . . . you are there . . . . in this beautiful iridescent white light . . . there with 'all that is' 'Creator of All That Is' . . . feelings of warmth flow through every cell of your body . . . enjoy those feelings . . . of unconditional love flowing through every cell of your body . . . remember that you are part of all that is . . . feel that connection now . . . .

If you see anyone . . . then you need to go higher . . . . As there is just you with 'Creator of All That Is'

Now just relax and enjoy the space . . . then take a deep breath in . . . you're still part of that white iridescent light . . . connected . . . knowing that you are part of 'all that is' . . . take another deep breath . . . . relaxing . . . knowing . . . and allow yourself a moment to enjoy these feelings . . . of all that is . . .

And now make the commands in your head . . . and if this is your first meditation, just be in this space of unconditional love, with love flowing through every cell of your body . . .

And now I want you to bring your awareness back . . . connecting back to that beautiful crystal . . . and bringing the awareness back through you body . . . to your crown and and as your awareness returns . . . you feel the chair . . . you are back in your space . . . and you are safe . . . and come back opening your eyes . . . . .

BEGINNING OF THE HEALING DOWNLOADS

Now you have a way of connecting to 'Creator of All That Is' so you are now ready to move on to downloading healings. Let's begin with the first set of healing downloads.

The list below shows the key beliefs that you will need to start on the journey to achieve your ideal weight. You will need to muscle test each one to ensure that you hold these beliefs. If any of these beliefs test negative, then you will need to download the healing from 'Creator of All That Is'.

I believe in instant healing
I am deserving of healing
I know what it feels like to heal
I know that it is safe to heal
I am worthy of healing
I am ready to heal now
I know what unconditional love feels like
I am worthy of all the good things in life and know what it feels like
I am worthy of all the good things in life and know what it feels like
I am accepting of all healings today
I allow myself to be freed from all negative energies today
I allow myself to be free from negative thoughts for today
I am open to learning everyday for my highest and best good
I want to heal
I know the process of grief

I know it's safe to allow the process of grief
The famine is over
I have the overweight gene—if yes;
I know what it feels like to live without the overweight
Gene
It's safe to release the overweight gene

Just remember the steps that you need to take.

> Set the Macro with 'Creator of All That Is'
> Go to the 'Creator of All That Is' and ask that the healing be carried out. This should be done in your mind so that you stay in the Theta Brain Wave state and witness the healings taking place
> Use the muscle test to see that the healing has been successful

When asking for a healing to be carried out you 'command' that it is done by 'Creator of All That Is'. When you have connected with 'Creator of All That Is' use the following command:

> **"'Creator of All That Is.', it is commanded that I have all these beliefs instilled in me, teach it** (or however you set your Macro) **for my highest and best good and in the highest and best way' thank you it is done, it is done, it is done. Show me . . . ."**

BLOCKS WHEN CONNECTING TO 'CREATOR OF ALL THAT IS'

I have worked with people who have struggled to make the connection with 'Creator of All That Is' and they ask me why it is that they are unable to connect.

I know that we are always connected to Source Energy, but sometimes I have felt as if I was completely alone, especially when I was going through some tough times, such as when I was suffering from depression. It seemed like I was at such a low state. I could hardly feel at all. It was at times like this that I was unable to feel the connection—this was my block.

Another block to feeling the connection is through our past lives. I have done many past life regressions, which for me are a source of fun as well as enlightenment without going back to the drama of the story. During some of these regressions I've been able to find a reason as to why I've been unable to connect. An example of this was from a past life where I had been persecuted and killed for being a healer. This gave me a subconscious belief that God had abandoned me. Healing this block enabled me to feel the connection and continue my journey.

A quick look at history shows us that life was often hard and it is therefore quite reasonable to assume that many of us have had difficult past lives. Another assumption that we can easily make is that many of us will have suffered persecution or religious prejudice. Subconsciously, you may relate these past life traumas to God, and may hold beliefs that Source Energy has abandoned you and you may still be holding anger within.

Being connected to 'Creator of All That Is' or Source Energy is in itself a source of nourishment, for it is the ultimate love, so it is possible to remove these blocks and experience that connection on deeper levels.

If you are struggling to connect to 'Creator of All That Is' it is good to test a few of these blocks, as well as any other blocks or scenarios that may spring to mind when thinking about them.

Using Muscle Testing and the process to download healings that you used in the previous section, you can test for the beliefs that may be blocking you. When testing for these beliefs, remember that I use the term God, you can use the Source Energy, Universal energy or whatever feels right for you!

> God abandoned me
> I am angry at God
> I am angry at God for . . . .
> God turned his back on me
> It is safe to connect to God

If you have any negative beliefs it would be a good idea to clear the issue first by connecting and using the following command. Remember that you could set a Macro to help you simplify the healing.

> **'Creator of All That Is . . . . It is commanded that I have the highest truth of the situation of** (when God abandoned me, or God turned his back on me) **I forgive myself, I forgive God, I ask that all anger and/ or resentments be lifted for my highest and best good, without creating grudges, all pain, shock and trauma is removed from me and I am healed from this situation completely and in the highest and best way, thank you, it is done, it is done, it is done . . . . Please show me'.**

When you have done this, remember that you need to use your mind's eye to witness the healing taking place.

The list of beliefs shown below are ones that I have seen remove blocks to connecting to 'Creator of All That Is', and you may want to test them to make sure that you have them. As always, you can use the name that most suits you when checking these.

I am connected to 'Creator of All That Is' . . .
'Creator of All That Is' is connected to me
'Creator of All That Is' is the light in which I see
I see myself as 'Creator of All That Is' sees me
I have 'Creator of All That Is' love with me always
I have the truth of 'Creator of All That Is'
'Creator of All That Is' is connected to me always
I am connected to 'Creator of All That Is' always
I am worthy of 'Creator of All That Is' love
I have proven myself to 'Creator of All That Is'
I am worthy of 'Creator of All That Is', of his love
It's safe to defend myself
God's love nourishes me

RESPONSIBILITY AND FORGIVENESS

If I believe that my thoughts create my life and everything to do with it, then it is time for me to take full responsibility for my life and be accepting of it. Yes, knowing that I have attracted everything that has happened to me and am fully responsible for it is a key acknowledgement when trying to resolve issues.

It is sometimes difficult to really accept the things that have happened to us, especially the traumatic experiences. However, being accepting of our life and all that goes with it is how we can begin to move forward.

Experiences come to us for all sorts of reasons; we could have learned something key from the situation or in some way the experience could be serving us. No matter what the reasons are for the experience manifesting itself, we must take full responsibility for it.

This was apparent in my relationships. I had many failed attempts at establishing a sound and lasting relationship, including two marriages. It was only when I finally took full responsibility for my life that I was able to see that I was attracting the same situations and the same type of relationships. The question that I now needed to answer was, "What did I need to learn from these events? "

I was not yet able to understand what I was learning from this continual cycle of events, as this lesson came to me before I found Theta healing and my connection to Source energy. But I did decide to take positive steps to break out of it. I asked my guides to help me, teach me the lessons I needed to learn in another way; following a repeated dream night after night I finally understood the lessons I needed to learn from my continual cycle of unhealthy relationships. I had the right to choose who I wanted to be with; I had the right to choose a person that could fulfil all my wishes and dreams in a relationship. I had the freedom of choice and worthy of that choice. So finally knew what I was learning from my past relationships and I could now be free and move on. From this point in my life, I never had another boyfriend or sought another relationship until I met my most compatible soul mate.

I also realised that, if I created every event in my life, and I was responsible for it then it was time to let go of blame.

It was also at this point that the realisation dawned on me that it was time to forgive all those who, in my eyes, had hurt me or stopped me achieving something. It was this realisation that enabled me to forgive them and, through forgiveness, I was able to release anger, hatred and even revenge.

Therefore, to be able to move on, you need to realise and believe that it is time to have compassion and forgiveness, compassion and forgiveness for everyone that has been involved in these cycles and that includes having compassion for and being able to forgive yourself!

If you can free your mind from negative emotions, you will free your body from the excess weight!

A lot of the excess weight in your body can be caused by you holding negative emotions and, therefore, if you are able to free yourself from these then you will be able to free your body form the excess weight. The following is a short exercise that will help you find and clear any negative emotions that you may well be holding on to. This may well be an ongoing process as your subconscious mind throws up thoughts and feelings. Listen carefully and, if you can hear where your mind is wandering, you may find new areas of your life that still need healing.

> ➤ Write a list of all the people you need to forgive or feel angry at
> ➤ Even if you don't know how to forgive, state that you are willing to forgive
> ➤ Remember to use the muscle test to confirm your feelings. It's amazing what you still may be holding in your subconscious mind, even your conscious mind might be telling you that you had moved on.
> ➤ You may want to do the download exercise first

If you are struggling as to how you need to express yourself in this area, then I have listed some examples below. If you need to, just use these and adapt them so that they feel right for you. This is not an exhaustive list just a few that may help you generate your own thoughts and beliefs.

> I am angry at myself for failing to . . . . .
> I am angry at [George] for hurting me
> I am angry at my father for . . . . .
> I am angry at [George] for . . . . .
> I truly forgive myself for . . . . ..
> I forgive [George] for hurting me
> I no longer resent [George] as I truly forgive them
> I am no longer angry at [George] as I truly forgive them

As you start to follow this process, it is a time to be very truthful with yourself. In my life, I have not always done things that I am proud of but, I am human, and I have allowed my human side and ego to get carried away with the stories and the drama. To be able to heal properly and start getting rid of my negative emotions, I needed to address all the areas of my life to help me be free from guilt. This can be achieved by using the following examples:

> I ask [George] to forgive me for . . . . ..
> I ask forgiveness for . . . . ..

Remember that you must always be able to forgive yourself for what you think you have done or not done. This gives you the ability to absolve yourself of all your subconscious guilt and start the process of shedding your negative emotions.

Once you have established what guilt, anger, pain or resentment you are holding, then you can use the Theta healing techniques we practiced earlier to connect with 'Creator of All That Is' and make the following statement for every scenario that requires healing:

> 'Creator of All That Is'; It is commanded that I have the highest truth of the situation, I forgive myself, I forgive **[George]**. I ask that all anger and/or resentment be lifted for my highest and best good, without creating grudges; that all pain, shock and trauma is removed from me and I am healed from this situation completely. Thank you, it is done, it is done, it is done . . . . Please show me'.

You can then use your mind's eye or your imagination to witness the healing taking place.

To see if you have the right beliefs to move forwards with compassion and forgiveness I suggest that, using the muscle test, you try testing the following beliefs. These and similar tests can be used for any area of your life that needs healing. If there are any beliefs that give a negative response, use the download and Macro process you learnt earlier to create the positive beliefs.

I have Creators truth of forgiveness
I know how to, and I do forgive myself
I know how to, and I do forgive others
I know how to have compassion for myself
I know how to have compassion for others
I forgive myself completely
I accept myself completely

I have creator's truth of my responsibilities for my life
I am responsible for my life
I accept responsibility for my life
I know when to recognise situations that need forgiveness
I know it is safe to forgive and move on now
I know how to live in the now and let go of past hurts
I know how to live in the now, this very moment this very second
I continue to forgive
I am accepting of all people and where they are in their life
I am willing to give up holding onto resentment
I let go of Guilt
I know how to live without Guilt
I know how to live without Shame
I (insert your name) no longer use food to punish myself
I know how to live without worry
I know how to live without anger
I have God's truth of revenge

We go through life with so many things to deal with. Sometimes we do not always give the time to heal from situations and we may be holding onto various feelings and emotions within our body. Ensure you test each one to see if you are holding any negative feelings, using the following example:

I am holding onto Stress

If this tests as a Yes, then use the healing technique

> "'Creator of All That Is', it is commanded that I have the highest truth of the situation, that created the stress, I forgive myself, I forgive all involved, I ask that I know how to live without stress, and all the stress held within me is sent to God's light and replaced with creators choice, and I am healed from this situation completely. Thank you, it is done, it is done, it is done . . . . Please show me"

If you are not holding stress, you may still want to confirm that
I know how to live without stress
I know how to live without pain
I know how to live without anxiety
I know how to live without criticism
I know how to live without anger
I know how to live without resentment
I release all resentment
I know how to live without sadness
I know how to live without hurt
I know how to live without being abused
I know how to live without being taken for granted
I know how to live without obsessions
I know how to live without depression
I know how to live without being ignored
I know how to live without being rejected
I know how to live without being abandoned
I know how to live without being overwhelmed or overstressed
I know what it feels like to live without regret
I know how to live without feeling lonely
I am free from regret

LOVING AND ACCEPTING OURSELVES

One of the key lessons that I've learnt with Theta healing is that "you are what you think". This automatically leads on to the powerful mantra that, if you are what you think, then by changing your thoughts you can change your life!

This shows the power of thought, which has been widely discussed in books about Theta healing as well as Louise Hay's Affirmations, The Secret and many other books. Even Rene Descartes, dubbed 'the Father of Modern Philosophy' is renowned for his statement "I think, therefore I am".

Bearing in mind just how powerful thought can be, this is an area that you can focus on to help achieve your ideal weight!

If I wake up in a positive mood, making statements like 'I'll have a great productive day today', I usually do. Likewise, if I wake up thinking that I feel awful and will have a terrible day, then the chances are quite strong that I will indeed have a bad day. Whenever you're not feeling 100%, try making positive statements—say them out loud! When I do this myself, just saying them makes me feel good. Try it yourself and see the difference it brings.

Our thoughts have substance . . . we think we are . . . .

Every thought that you think starts out psychically, but then returns to you in a physical manifestation. Whether it is a person, a thing, a condition or a circumstance. Therefore if you choose your thoughts you choose your life.

How do we really feel and speak about our bodies?

So many of us go through our lives with statements like

I hate my legs . . . . I'm too fat . . . . .

I remember when I was younger; I always wore a cardigan to hide my shapely curves, as I felt they were too shapely.

You are aware of your own thoughts and feelings about your body even though you may not realise it today, so tune in to it and listen to yourself.

If you have negative thoughts about your body, change that today. In the list below you fill find a list of beliefs that you can test against to help you have the right beliefs to being loved and accepting yourself 'just as you are'.

Using the download and Macro techniques you learnt earlier, test yourself for these beliefs and change any that may give a negative response. As you're doing this exercise, you may find other thoughts coming to mind. If you do, just add them to the list and carry on testing.

I know how to and I do like my body
I know how to and I do, love myself
The more I like my body the more I love my body
I accept myself for who I am
I accept and understand my body
I know how to listen to my body
I value myself and my body
I live my life fully accepting of my body
I know how to take care of my body
I know how to pamper and support my body
I know how to pleasure my body
I know how to recognise how beautiful my body is

My body is beautiful
I know how to recognise how strong my body is
I know how to respect my body
I forgive my body
My body forgives me
I am kind to myself and my body
I trust my body
My body trusts me

DEALING WITH OUR FEELINGS AND EMOTIONS

Do we really understand our feelings and emotions?

Do we hide or bury them?

I remember eating a fried egg sandwich, thick white bread and drinking a large cup of tea with it but still feeling empty. Listening to myself, and muscle testing I realised I wasn't hungry for food, but I was hungry for affection.

Our subconscious feelings and emotions can have a great affect on our eating habits and our "need" for sustenance, so being able to recognise these and change them for the better is a key area in your journey to achieving your ideal weight.

From personal experience, I know it took approximately 8 years for me to fully accept losing my mother to cancer. I felt cheated, angry and had all sorts of emotions that I didn't know how to deal with. Burying emotions really affects us physically and emotionally, if we can really deal with our emotions in the right way, we become free. During these 8 years I struggled with my weight and wasted time, effort and money on various diets that simply didn't work.

Can you recognise if you eat because you feel lonely or bored?

Are you an emotional eater?

Can you recognise that the hunger you feel is not for food, but for the easing of an emotion or feeling?

You can use the following list of beliefs to establish where you may be holding negative feelings and emotions that are preventing you from achieving your ideal weight. Using the download and Macro techniques you learnt earlier, test yourself for these beliefs and change any that may give a negative response. As you're doing this exercise, you may find other thoughts coming to mind. If you do, just add them to the list and carry on testing.

I have Creator's truth of what my feelings and emotions are

It is safe to feel my feelings and emotions

I am able to feel my feelings and emotions

I know how to welcome my emotions and feelings with tenderness

I know what I really feel

I know how to relate to my feeling and emotions

I trust what my feelings and emotions are saying

I know how to deal with my feelings and emotions for my highest good

I know how to deal with my feelings and emotions without turning to food

I know how to live without retreating from my feelings and emotions

I know how to recognise the situations that are affecting my emotions

I know how to deal with my feelings and emotions without harming my body

I know how to deal with my anger in the highest and best way for me

I know how to deal with my feelings and emotions in the highest and best way for all

I know how to live without emotionally eating

I know how to live without eating out of boredom

I know how to live without eating out of loneliness

I know how to eat only when I am hungry for food

I know how to live without eating to please others
I know how to live without eating to prove anything to others
I know how to live without eating to fit in
I know how to live without feeling empty

I know what Joy feels like
I know what Happiness feels like
I know what it feels like to have comfort
I know what it feels like to belong
I know what it feels like to Trust others
I know what it feels like to Relax
I know what it feels like to have Courage
I know what it feels like to Say No
I know what it feels like to feel Safe
I know what it feels like to Be Heard
I know what it feels like to feel Whole
I know what it feels like to be Calm
I know what it feels like to feel Contented
I know what it feels like to be Listened To
I know what it feels like to be Heard
I know what it feels like to be Understood by others
I know what it feels like to be Nurtured
I know what it feels like to feel Wanted
I know what it feels like to feel Cherished

INNER CHILD

Wikipedia defines the Inner Child as being

"A concept used in popular psychology and Analytical psychology to denote the childlike aspect of a person's psyche, especially when viewed as an independent entity".

Wiktionary defines it as being:

> *"The essential, or original self, regarded as a child, existing within the shell of an adult, especially when suppressed by negative childhood experiences"*

The first time I connected to my inner child was during my Hypnotherapy and Psychotherapy training. It was a real moving experience as I saw some of the emotions my inner child was holding on to. She was a very angry little girl and I realised that any situation in my life that involved anger had the fury from this little girl attached to it.

Your inner child is another part of you that will enlighten you to any suppressed negative experiences, and this will enhance your journey to achieve your ideal weight. Being able to readily see and understand these suppressed negative experiences shows you what we need to heal.

It's also the fun child part of us and helps give us the naïve joy and wonder of a child through which we can enjoy life more.

You can use a meditation to connect to your Inner Child but, before you try this, I would suggest reviewing the list below and use the download techniques you learnt earlier to change any negative responses.

> I have creator's truth and understanding of my inner child
> I know how to connect to my inner child
> I know how to take care of my inner child
> I know how to communicate with my inner child

INNER CHILD MEDITATION

This is a meditation that will help you connect to your Inner Child. Before attempting this meditation please refer back to point 2 in the section "How to Use this Book to do Your Own Healing Downloads" to refresh your memory as to the best way for you to work through it.

Close your eyes . . . and take a deep breath . . . breath deeper and deeper . . . . Allow your mind to settle . . . . just relax . . . you relax . . . more and more . . . allowing yourself to just . . . focus . . . focus on the sound of these words . . . focusing and relaxing . . . knowing that you have been in a relaxed state before and that you can easily find those feelings of complete calm . . . and you can find those feelings of complete relaxation . . . easily and effortlessly . . . allowing the body to relax as you sink into the chair . . . . Allowing your mind to relax . . . with each and every breath you take . . . relaxing more . . .

Where total tranquillity awaits . . . you find your mind wandering to a place . . . it's a place you know . . . or it's imaginary . . . but it's your place . . . a place to feel safe and secure . . . a place to relax . . . a place to relax in your mind . . . and your body . . . and as you relax even more . . . you feel that sense of calmness washing all over you . . . in your safe and secure place . . . . just for you . . . . there may be sounds . . . . or it may be silent . . . .

What can you see?

What colours or shapes are around you?

It's your unique place to just relax and let go . . . it may be warm or slightly cool but whatever it is . . . it is just right for you . . . it maybe indoors or outdoors . . . there may be smells . . . or the sound of the breeze whistling through the trees . . . it all reminds you . . . of how safe and secure you are . . . in this relaxed unique place . . . .

Now give your place a name . . . . a name that is unique to you . . . .

So whenever you need a time of relaxation and calm . . . . you will just have say the name . . . . close your eyes and all these feelings of deep relaxation and calmness will return to you . . . . .

While you are in this beautiful protected space . . . I want you to meet someone very special . . . . and very close to you . . . someone who is within you always . . . .

A little girl or boy . . . inside of you . . . your inner child . . . .

Look and see this beautiful inner child within you . . . . always there . . . . always part of you . . . . the emotional you . . . the fun part of you . . . . part of you . . . .

Are they close to you . . . or somewhere in the distance? Wherever they are they are close to you . . .

Ask if they would like to talk to you . . . see if there is something they wish to say . . . take this time to hear your inner child . . . . . .

You may want to know their name . . . or you may already know it . . . . is there something you would like to say to them?

You know what your inner child needs to hear . . . maybe speak to them now . . . give them a few moments to respond . . . listen . . . listen . . . listen to what they have to say back to you . . .

It's time to understand your inner child . . . acknowledge and embrace them . . . and listen to them . . . . take time to hear . . . . . . have this time to really get to know your inner child . . . and thank them . . . thank them for guiding you through life with emotions even if you were not able to listen . . . ..

I'll give you a few moments . . . . a few moments to get to know and understand your inner child . . . .

You feel it's time to embrace your inner child . . . . Bring that beautiful inner child to you . . .

That's it . . . connect . . . . And thank your inner child . . . .

And in this safe space . . .

Take another deep breath . . . . Relaxing . . . . and now I want you to bring your awareness back to your body . . . .

Knowing that you have given yourself . . . this day . . . this day to heal . . . and you have received some beautiful healings and tools to create in your life whatever it is you wish . . .

And you are ready to enjoy the journey of healing . . . remembering your safe unique place full of relaxation . . . and feelings of calm anytime you need it . . . now

You feel your body . . . . you feel the chair . . . you are back in your space . . . your feet are back on the ground . . . and you are safe . . . you return to the room

BELIEVE YOURSELF TO YOUR IDEAL WEIGHT

As you saw in the section on Loving and Accepting Ourselves, our thoughts and beliefs are extremely powerful.
We really are our beliefs . . .

I've spoken to people who constantly maintain their ideal weight and they tell me they can eat whatever they like without putting on any weight. What a tremendous belief to hold!

If you think of how many people have been told they are exactly like their mother, and then end up looking just like their mother! In fact, one of the beliefs that I once held was that when I get to over 40 I will put on weight and it will be very difficult to reduce. I had been told this so many times that I actually believed it and, guess what? When I reached 40 that is exactly what has happened to me!

In the pharmaceutical world, people on drug trials are often given the placebo rather than the actual drug and, in some cases, they actually become well. Just by believing that the "medication" they have been given will cure them, they actually become better.

You can develop a similar effect by continually making new statements that, if said enough times will become beliefs and will then manifest themselves in your life. These are called 'Affirmations' and are especially prevalent in eastern religions and belief systems such as Buddhism.

We are made up of many subconscious beliefs, so it is important that, as we go forward, we truly believe that we are our ideal weight.

That way, we can achieve and always maintain our ideal weight as well as manifesting many more new beliefs and feelings

As you go forward always remember the power of your spoken words and thoughts. If you continually state 'I need to lose weight' there will be two affects. Firstly, you may always **"needing to"** and secondly, as we all know, if you lose something, you will search for a long time until you find it again. So rather than thinking and talking about 'losing' weight, change your words to 'reducing' weight or 'achieving your ideal weight'. This simple change of wording can have a massive affect on your beliefs and your life!

Remember the power of our thoughts . . .

Now we get to some of the key areas and beliefs that really affect the amount of weight that you carry. With the following downloads you will be able to ascertain what your ideal weight is and if you have the right beliefs in your subconscious to be able to achieve it.

Using the download and Macro techniques you learnt earlier in the book, test the following key beliefs and, if need be ask 'Creator of All That Is' to give you them:

I have Creators truth, perspective and understanding of my ideal body composition

I have Creators truth, perspective and understanding of my weight set point

Once you have the above downloads testing positively, you can now use the muscle testing technique to establish what your ideal weight is.

Start at a weight that you feel happy with, using stones and pounds or kilograms, whichever the units are that you will be using to measure your weight (I will be using stones (st) and pounds (lbs) in the examples that I give).

For example:

> My ideal weight is 9st = No
> My ideal weight 8st 9lbs = No
> My ideal weight is 8st 4lbs = Yes
> In this example, your ideal weight would be 8st 4lbs, so you would then ask 'Creator of All That Is' to teach you that you are 8st 4lbs.

Remember, you have a choice to be whatever you wish so, if you choose to be 9st then you will be 9st!

Once you have established what your ideal weight is, then you can start to work on the beliefs that will help or hinder you achieving your ideal weight.

Again, using the muscle test, with the download and Macro techniques you learnt earlier in the book, test yourself for the following beliefs and, if any give a negative response, ask 'Creator of All That Is' to change the belief to be positive. As in previous exercises, listen to your subconscious and, if any other beliefs spring to mind, then test for them as well.

> I am . . . . .. (enter your ideal body weight or your weight set point)
> I achieve and maintain my ideal body composition, from 'Creator's' perspective
> I can reduce my weight until I achieve my ideal body weight
> I choose the right foods to enhance my weight reduction
> I choose the right foods to maintain a healthy body
> I can eat whatever I choose and maintain my ideal weight
> I have 'Creators' truth of all the times I previously dieted
> I have 'Creators' truth of dieting

Everything I eat brings me health and happiness
I process all the food I eat
I can eat without storing excess fat
I do release excess fat with grace and ease
I process and draw nutrition from all foods
I understand the right work life balance from Creator's perspective
I can eat excess fat without storing it in my body
I am deserving of being *use your ideal weight*
I am worthy of being *use your ideal weight*
It is safe to be *use your ideal weight*
It is safe to be perfect
I am perfect at *use your ideal weight*
My body co-operates to maintain my ideal weight
I am *use your ideal weight* without counting calories
I am *use your ideal weight* without dieting
I see myself at *use your ideal weight*
I know what it feels like to be *use your ideal weight*
I tell my body everyday how beautiful it is being and feeling *use your ideal weight*
Food does not hurt me, unless I believe it will
My body reduces weight daily until I reach *use your ideal weight*

ADDITIONAL FACTS

pH Balance

In recent years, there has been a growing belief that the acidic/alkaline balance of the body can have a great impact on our health and that, if we maintain the correct balance, it can lead to significantly better health, improving our immunity and slowing down the ageing process.

A good dietary balance is to have at least 80% alkalizing foods & 20% of neutral and acidifying foods.

Eating more raw foods will increase your alkaline balance or you can also find Alkalising Drops and Jugs that will increase the alkaline level in water. By drinking this water (but not to excess) you can increase the alkaline level of your body.

As part of her Theta teaching, Vianna Stibal, the founder of Theta healing teaches that alkaline foods make the body uninhabitable to parasites, bacteria, viruses, fungi and other microbes. Therefore, the closer to the ideal acid/alkaline balance (known as the pH balance) we get our bodies to, the less likely we are to be affected by these, and the healthier we will be.

The ideal pH balance is in the range of 7.2—7.4 and, if you search the internet, you will be able to find more information about this, as well as various food charts that will give you the acidic or alkaline value of key food products.

There are also many who believe that, the more positive a person is, the more alkaline the body is and, the more negative a person is, the more acidic the body is. So changing subconscious negative beliefs will improve your acid/alkaline balance!

It is not important to understand any of the chemistry around the pH balance to be healthy, reduce your weight, or do great Theta healing but, for the curious, Wikipedia defines pH as:

> *"pH is a measure of the acidity or alkalinity of a solution.*
>
> *Aqueous solutions at 25°C with a pH less than seven are considered acidic, while those with a pH greater than seven are considered basic (alkaline).*
>
> *When a pH level is 7.0, it is defined as 'neutral' at 25°C because at this pH the concentration of H3O + equals the concentration of OH − in pure water.*
>
> *pH is formally dependent upon the activity of hydronium ions (H3O+), but for very dilute solutions, the molarity of H3O+ may be used as a substitute with little loss of accuracy. (H+ is often used as a synonym for H3O+.)"*

There is a very simple way to test your pH balance, and you will need some pH strips (which can be bought very cheaply on the internet). The exact instructions on how to test your pH balance will come with the strips but basically the simple test is as follows:

Wait at least 2 hours after eating. Fill your mouth with saliva and then swallow it. Do this again to help ensure that the saliva is clean. Then the third time put some saliva onto pH paper.

Compare the colour with the chart that comes with the pH paper. If your saliva is acid (below pH of 7.0) wait two hours and repeat the test.

Water

Every single living cell is made up of **water** (intracellular fluid) and surrounded by water (extra cellular fluid). Every one of our tissues and sustaining processes requires water to function properly, which includes the release of excess fat, flushing out toxins, and the chemical reaction that breaks down the fat itself. Therefore, to help us reduce our weight and achieve our ideal weight, it is essential that we drink plenty of water, but not too much!

Food Intolerances

Some of us suffer from **food intolerances**, and this can have an effect on our energy levels. We may crave high energy foods to keep going and this, in turn, will have an effect on the amount of weight we carry.

Theta can be used to heal in all areas of our lives, and food allergies are no exception. We can heal allergies using Theta as long as we can get down to the bottom belief.

It would be impossible to address all the possible allergies in this book so for today we will ask to process the more common allergies with grace and ease.

As in all the previous exercises, you use the muscle testing technique along with the download and Macro techniques to test the following beliefs and, where necessary, ask 'Creator of All That Is' to change the negative ones back into positive ones. Of course, if you have any food intolerances, then you can add them to the list and ask for them to be healed.

> I know the difference between hunger and thirst
> I like water
> I know how to stay slightly alkaline

My body processes wheat with grace and ease
My body processes dairy with grace and ease
My body processes sugar with grace and ease
My body processes wheat gluten with grace and ease
My body increases its Basal Metabolic Rate that is for my highest good
I know how live without being addicted to sugar

INTIMACY AND RELATIONSHIPS

In our lives we all have many experiences, some we really enjoy and some we would not have wished for. Whatever beliefs or traumas we may hold and for whatever reason, be they from this lifetime, a past life, a belief from our ancestors or on a soul level, we can heal and change them.

I remember a time when I was 30 years old and single (with two wonderful children). I was looking good, feeling good, quite attractive, and gained much attention from men. However, I soon realised that the attention was not always for what I call a genuine relationship, more like 'lets have some fun', which definitely wasn't what I was looking for. At this time I remember swearing that I no longer wish to be attractive as I will never know if someone wants me for me, or just for 'a bit of fun'.

I realise now that I have the strength and am happy to say 'no' to anyone that asks for anymore of me than I am prepared to give.

So it is important we check this area of our life, and if I Swore I actually made an Oath to myself, never to be attractive and slim again!

I have come across Oaths, Vows, Curses and Commitments that have been preventing me becoming all I wish to be, so it's good to check.

You could be holding a curse that has been handed down from generations; an ancestor may have accepted it and handed it down to you through the generations. Another type of curse is what we know about from older generation's voodoos, for example, the Greeks or the Romans. However, you would only accept the curse if you are holding guilt or fear or some other negative emotions.

I visited Roman Baths to find a pool full of curses. At the time of the Romans, it seems that if someone did wrong to you, then the thing to do was to write the curse down and throw it into the pool. If you believed in this as a way of payback, then you would have accepted it.

If we make an Oath or Vow it is a statement of fact, and you may call upon something sacred, such as a bible or 'as God is my witness'. It binds us on a deeper level.

Some examples of vows that you may hold are vows of poverty, chastity, sacrifice, punishment, never to love, subservience, silence, martyrdom, or celibacy.

So ask yourself:

Is your excess weight protecting you from unwanted attention?
Is your excess weight protecting you physically and/or emotionally?
Are you carrying excess weight for fear of intimacy?
Are there past events that are still affecting you now?

To see if you are holding any oaths or vows that might be affecting the amount of weight you are carrying, muscle test the following:

My excess weight is protecting me
I fear intimacy
My fat keeps me safe
I have oaths, vows, curses or commitments preventing me being my ideal weight
I have oaths, vows, curses or commitments preventing me being successful

➤ If you can muscle test the Oaths, Vows, Curses, Commitments or Contracts, from above (remember to use clear statements and not ask questions) then you will need to try and establish what they are. Below are some examples that you may wish to test on. Of course, if you feel that there are others that you are carrying then test them as well.

I have a vow of celibacy
I have a vow of silence
I am cursed never to love etc . . .
I swore to hold onto excess weight

➤ If, after two or three attempts, you have downloads from any section that do not change, check to see if they are being held in by an Oath, Vow, Curse, Commitment or Contract.

➤ Remember these are all beliefs, try not be caught up in any drama of past lives, just heal the issue and move on.

➤ If you still have issues ask yourself:

It serves me to have a vow of celibacy
I am learning from this vow of celibacy

If you tested yes, then think (and muscle test) to find out what it is, for example:

I am learning to value my own body by this vow of celibacy.
I am learning to be independent by remaining celibate.

Once you have what you need, you can add them to your download list—

I know how to value my own body
I know how *to be independent without being celibate.*

If you find that you are carrying Oaths, Vows, Curses, Commitments or Contracts then use the example below (this one is for Curses) to get rid of them:

> *'Creator of All That Is' it is commanded that the Curse that . . . . Is removed from me, from all that I am, it is completed and no longer needed, thank you it is done, it is done, it is done . . . show me.*

Watch in your mind's eye and witness the Curse being removed.

You may see the energy being removed from all the levels where the belief is held. You may be able to watch it being pushed out of your feet, as you imagine gathering it up to send up to God's light and never to return, being transformed into love and light.

For the rest the others, you may want to try the following:

> *'Creator of All That Is' it is commanded that the Vow (Oath, commitment or contract) of . . . (**put the details of it here**). It is removed from me, from all that I am. It is completed and no longer needed. Thank you it is done, it is done, it is done . . . show me . . .*

You will see it being lifted and marked complete.

Below, I have given you some examples of other beliefs that, when tested negative, may influence the amount of weight that you carry, and prevent you achieving your ideal weight.

Using the download and Macro exercises, test each one and, where necessary, ask 'Creator of All That Is' to change the belief to be positive.

> It is safe to release excess weight
> I can let go of fear and allow 'Creator of All That Is' to guide me
> I have Creator's perspective, definition and understanding of Intimacy

I have Creator's perspective, definition and understanding of Love

I have Creator's perspective, definition and understanding of Soul mates

I have the discretion to know when it's in my best interest to be intimate

I know what it feels like to be safe with my most compatible soul mate/partner

I know how to be intimate with a man/woman

I know how to be intimate with a man/woman and be safe at the same time

I know how to be close to God and with a human partner at the same time

I know how to be loved by a companion

I know how to love people for who they are

I know what a partner's love feels like

I know what it feels like to have a mother's love

I know what it feels like to have a father's love

ARE WE GAINING FROM BEING OVERWEIGHT?

Another key area that can affect our ability to reduce our weight is to work out whether or not we are gaining from being overweight?

On my journey to achieving my ideal weight, I have uncovered many negative belief systems that were keeping my weight firmly in place. I was never quite good enough, I would never stand out, and I would never be perfect. You may need to meditate and allow your mind to wander to really uncover if you are gaining from being overweight.

You could ask 'I am learning from being overweight, or it serves me to be overweight, it's understanding what do we gain by being overweight.

I have given you an exercise below that will help you determine if you are gaining by being overweight:

Write a list of what you feel you may be gaining by being overweight

> It proves I am unworthy
  I have a reason for failing
  I have an excuse for this anger

> Reword them and add them to the download list
  I am worthy
  I live without fear of failure
  I forgive and let go of anger

> ➢ Also check
>> I am learning from being overweight
>> It serves me to be overweight

If you have tested 'yes' to any of these, you will need to find out how and why, and ask 'Creator of All That Is' to teach you how to. For example:

> If you have tested that 'I am learning to fully accept myself by being overweight'
> Then you will need to download 'I fully accept myself'.

You may find many other ways in which you are gaining form being overweight, and each one can be processed using the above example.

You can sue the following downloads to help understand more areas of why you may be holding on to excess weight:

I know what it feels like to know to live without being overweight or using food:

> to hide
> as a punishment
> to be Godly
> to bury emotions
> to prove I am unworthy
> for a diversion
> to replace love
> to find peace
> for fulfilment

And below you will find some more beliefs that you can use as examples to see which need to be changed to help you achieve your ideal weight.

> I am good enough
> I am worthy

I live without the fear of failing
I know the difference between comfort and food
I know the difference between love and food
I know how to enjoy food when I am hungry
I know what my body wants
I know what my body needs
Every time I feel hungry I can identify if it's for food
I know the difference between my emotions and food
Every time I'm hungry I can identify if it's for food or other emotions
I know how to identify what emotions are being triggered
I know how to find protection without using fat
I am safe in this world without having to have fat or to be fat
I know how to be safe without using fat
I can be abundant without being overweight
I know it's safe for me to be successful
I can achieve
I know how to live without over eating

CHILDHOOD BELIEFS

Although talked about a lot, and researched in many areas, the fact that we may still carry beliefs that originate from our childhood is often forgotten.

I was lucky as a child. We were never forced to finish our plate of food. I know it can be an issue when a child has had to finish every item on their plate or forced to eat food they never liked. I am sure our parents did it for all the right reasons, but it may have left some scars . . . .

Do you feel guilty if you leave your food? Were you told that there are children starving out there in the 3rd world who would be grateful of what you'd left on your plate?

Are you still carrying beliefs from your childhood that may be affecting you in achieving your goals?

Here is an exercise to help you see:

- ➤ Think about your own childhood, note down and muscle test what feels right for you and test the following examples
  I am guilty if I leave food on my plate
  It's wrong to leave food on your plate
  It's wrong to waste food

- ➤ Reword and create additional downloads
  I can eat until I am comfortable
  I have plenty
  I can eat until I am full without feeling guilty

I can enjoy the food I eat until I am satisfied
I have 'Creator's' truth and understanding of what
would happen if I left food on my plate

Using the following downloads and Macros, you will be able to see which beliefs may be hindering you:

I have 'Creator's' truth of what my parents/teachers have told me
I know how to stand up to my parents
I am loved and accepted by my parents no matter what I eat, even if I choose to leave food on my plate
I can choose what and when I want to eat without upsetting anyone
I am in control of what I eat and when
I put myself first without being selfish
I can eat what I choose to eat without feeling guilty
I know what it feels like to eat when I am hungry for food
I know what it feels like to eat sitting down in a calm environment. (This does not include the car).
I know what it feels like to eat without distractions. (Distractions include radio, television, newspapers, books, intense or anxiety-producing conversations or music).
I know what it feels like to eat what my body wants.
I know what it feels like to eat until I am satisfied.
I know what it feels like to eat (with the intention of being) in full view of others.
I know what it feels like to eat with enjoyment, gusto and pleasure.

PHYSICAL HEALING

Theta healing works on any area of your life. By uncovering the emotional reasons you have the condition it will promote and enhance any physical, emotional and spiritual issues. It is such a wonderful thing to do!

When using Theta to heal physical conditions, it is essential that you always continue with your health care and never stop any medication unless you are advised to do so by your Doctor.

If there is a deep rooted emotional issue that is causing the physical symptoms, then you can always seek the support of a qualified Theta Practitioner.

Below you will find some of the key areas that have been found to address this area in relation to retaining excess weight.

Use the meditation to 'Creator of All That Is' and make the command for each one to be done in the highest and best way for your highest good . . . . thank you, it is done, it is done, show me . . .

Work on them one by one, and ensure that you watch them to completion.

> Increase BMR for your highest good at this time
> Activate your Youth and Vitality Gene
> Activate your DNA
> Remove free Radicals from your body
> Remove excess Radiation from your body
> Remove Mercury Poisoning from your body

Regenerate any cells for their highest and best good
Regenerate skin elasticity
Balance all hormone levels for your highest good

You can ask 'Creator of All That Is' to do a physical healing on any area of your body. If the healing is not permanent and the ailment comes back, you can ask Creator, if you are learning from it, or how is it serving you. Use the muscle test to check your subconscious beliefs.

BEING YOUR IDEAL WEIGHT

Today we constantly hear about people wanting to lose weight or wanting to reduce weight, but what is it that we are really trying to achieve? When will we know when we have "lost" enough weight or "reduced" our weight sufficiently? How can we tell that we really are carrying excess weight?

As everyone is different and the ways our bodies are built are unique, it is almost impossible to answer any of these questions. To me, the whole point of focussing on our weight is to achieve our "Ideal Weight". Again, how do we know what our ideal weight is? You can read many magazines, articles and books that will tell you, depending on your body type, age and sex, what your supposed ideal weight should be. As you have seen in a previous exercise, we can use our subconscious to determine what our ideal weight is.

This exercise is here to identify any other blocks to being your ideal weight that you may hold. You can use it more than once; keep going until it feels real to be at your perfect weight and size.

You may see people or emotions that are preventing you from being your ideal weight.

When doing this exercise, I discovered that if I got to my ideal weight people would say I look gaunt and sick. So I associated reducing my weight with being sick. To combat this belief, I created the following downloads

I can be my ideal weight without looking gaunt
I can be my ideal weight without being ill or sick
I can be my ideal weight and be healthy

Do you know how good it feels to be your ideal weight? To help you experience this, I have developed the following meditation. Remember that you can do the meditation in the way that is best for you, reading it yourself, recording it so that you can play bit back to yourself, or having a good friend read it to you.

I want you to take a deep breath in and relax . . . close your eyes and relax . . . . that's it . . . just relax . . . with every breath you take you relax deeper and deeper . . . .

And with every breath you take you relax deeper . . . . and feelings of warmth and comfort begin to surround you now . . . as you breathe deeper and deeper . . . and you begin to settle into a more relaxed state than before . . . .

You relax and let go . . . giving yourself this time, this space, this day . . . a day just for you . . . this is your time . . . . for you . . . .

Now relaxing every muscle in your body as you relax more and more . . . . You find your mind wandering . . . . drifting . . . relaxing . . . safe and secure . . . .

And I want you to just focus on the sound of my voice . . . .

And as you become relaxed you become more aware of your abilities that you have within you . . . . you become connected to that part of you that is comfortable and confident . . . .

You imagine yourself walking . . . walking on a clear beautiful day . . . the weather is just how you like it . . . neither too hot nor too cold, just perfect for you . . . .

You hear slight sounds in the distance . . . but none that disturb you . . . .

The colours in the sky . . . and the trees are so clear . . . . . so clear as if today . . . today you have so much clarity . . . you can see clearly . . . . and it's so beautiful . . . you are filled with warmth, and joy . . . a warmth a joy that you remember feeling before . . .

And as you walk you notice how you are feeling . . . . you begin to feel slightly different than before . . . with the same warmth and joy . . . but now you feel and see yourself at your ideal body weight . . . the ideal weight that's just perfect for you . . .

See yourself at that perfect weight now . . . . .

How does it feel?

How comfortable do you feel?

Keep walking . . . experience all those feelings . . . just walk and take note of all that you are feeling now . . . .

Think of others that are in your lives . . . how do they look to you now? Now you're at your ideal weight . . . as you walk you learn . . . what you need to learn . . . for this journey is a journey of discovery . . . each step you take brings you more awareness of who you are . . . .

Keep walking . . . feeling . . . .

Learning . . . . .

Now . . . remembering all what you have learnt and felt on your journey . . . Come back . . . refreshed and alert

After you have completed the meditation, try answering the following questions:

How did that feel being at your perfect weight?
Did it feel as you imagined?
What are you doing when it's gone?
Did it feel as you imagined?
Was there anything preventing you?
Was there anyone preventing you?

➢ If you found some feelings, or maybe recognised a block, then, using the appropriate downloads and Macros, go through the healing process:
I am like mother
I am afraid of success

➢ Reword and Download the above to read:
I can be like my mother without being overweight
It's safe to be successful

SPIRIT GUIDES AND GUARDIAN ANGELS

So many people forget to engage with their Spirit Guides and Guardian Angels. Their purpose is to guide and protect us.

I have asked my guides to help find the answers to so many questions; I have always been answered via a book, a dream, a whisper or just through my intuition. The only lesson that I had to learn was how to ask and how to listen for the answer. It is very simple, we just ask and we are heard.

We can ask them to help us heal from situations or physical conditions. They are there for us, so why not use this wonderful connection to move forward in any areas of our life. This is not just our ideal weight, but also with such things as a new job, a new house and many more areas of our lives.

Guardian Angels are with us always; if we have death door experiences they may change. Spirit Guides may come and go depending on what it is we need to learn at the time.

To read up on Spirit Guides, Guardian Angles and Ascended Masters you can find many articles and books out there on the market; there are so many ways to find help, support and answers to our questions.

For me my own Spirit Guides and Guardian Angels are an endless source of help and guidance . . . I just have to ask!

If you end these exercises and there are still issues with your weight, you can ask 'Creator of All That Is' or your spirit guides and guardian angels to help find the answers that you need to find for you.

The following as a list of beliefs that, using the download and Macro process, you will be able to test to see how connected you are to your Spirit Guides and Guardian Angels.

I have Creators truth of my Spirit Guides and Guardian Angels

I am connected to my Spirit Guides and Guardian Angels

My Spirit Guides and Guardian Angels are connected to me

I know how to ask my Spirit Guides and Guardian Angels for guidance

I know how to fully communicate to my Spirit Guides and Guardian Angels

I know the difference between their voice and my voice

I know how to trust my intuition

I know my true self

I know what it feels like to know my true self

I know it is possible for me to know my life purpose

I know my life purpose

I know the next steps to take for my highest good

I know how to make the choices in alignment for my highest purpose

I know how to recognise the people to be with that serve my highest purpose

I know how to manifest all that I desire in my life

HEALTHY LIFESTYLE

Up until now, we have focused on the spiritual barriers that you may have preventing you from achieving your ideal weight. However, it is essential that you have, and maintain a healthy lifestyle.

This section is about creating a healthy lifestyle to move on with as well as providing you with some healing downloads to heal your mind and body, and create well being.

I always use the muscle testing technique to decide questions I am not sure of. If people tell me that going on a detox diet is a good thing I muscle test to confirm if this is the case for me. I just say:

> 'It is for my highest good to go on a detox diet'. In my case, this inevitably answered with a 'No!' (Phew!!)

There was one time that my subconscious told me that I did need to go on a detox diet but I only needed it for 7 days.

Always remember to always ask for Creator's truth and understanding of the particular detox diet, and that your truth is the same as his. Examples of this are:

> It is for my highest good to go on a diet = No
> It is for my highest good to eat healthy nourishing foods = Yes

You can also use this technique to dig deeper and break it down to the types of food that are or aren't good for you to eat at the particular point in time.

It is for my highest good to eat red meats = Yes
It is for my highest good to eat fish = Yes

for whatever foods you wish to check for. Remember to state it is for my highest good to eat a portion of meat every day, or today, or now.

The more that you begin to understand your eating habits, you will find that additional beliefs come up that you can check and deal with.

I can eat healthy foods without binge eating. This is a belief that always returned a negative answer until I'd found it and changed it. When I test this now, I get a most definite 'YES!'

I now believe that I can eat whatever I want without putting on weight.

Although on this journey many beliefs were preventing me; One morning I felt very hungry after breakfast, I muscle tested I am hungry for food = No. I then tested I am empty = Yes. So I asked for a healing.

If we are truthful to ourselves, and really listen to our bodies, feelings, and with the help of the subconscious mind, using the muscle test as confirmation we can achieve our ideal weight now.

My conscious mind needed to know how to maintain my ideal weight as I don't remember a time in my life that my weight remained stable.

It's all down to our beliefs, and below you can find some areas that you can address with the download and Macro techniques:

Every day in every way I get healthier
I am healthy

I feel good about myself
I know how and when to relax
I am in perfect balance
I create the right balance in my life
I know how to and I do break the unhealthy habits in my life
I know how to and I do, deal with cravings in the best way, for my highest good
I can live in the present moment
I have the power to be my ideal weight
I can have miracles in my life
I can have happy endings
I can expect whatever I wish for
I do succeed
I am inspired to achieve
I can control my life
I can control what I eat
I know how to eat until I'm full
I know how to eat until satisfied
I know the reasons I turn to food
I understand the definition of eating right
I can live without constantly thinking about food
I know what it feels like to eat right
I know what it feels like to reduce in weight
I know how to reduce in weight
I have the confidence to change my life for my highest good
I have the commitment to change my life for my highest good
I know how to achieve and maintain my ideal weight
My faith grows more and more each day
If I get stuck I hand it over to 'Creator of All That Is'
I give thanks and bless all the food I eat

I integrate all these healings with grace and ease
I keep all these healings throughout this lifetime

A FINAL THOUGHT

The contents of this book were designed to be part of a one day workshop to help people to understand how subconscious thoughts and beliefs can affect our lives, and to help them on their journey to reduce the amount of weight they are carrying and to help them see the way to their ideal weight.

I have tried and tested all of the exercises in this book and I will continue to do so as it has been a journey of discovery for me.

It is a process where you can look closely within yourself and see what it is for you, why you hold excess weight and what it is for you that will help you change.

Remember the importance of getting the muscle testing right. Never ask a question, always make a statement such as 'It is for my highest good to eat vegetables today'.

If you find that you develop blocks to the healings check the following:

> If it is serving you, or are you learning from it?
> Test for Oaths, Vows, Curses, Commitments or Contracts
> Redo the exercises and use the muscle test to confirm you have healed
> If in doubt ask 'Creator of All That Is'
> If you come up with a block or fear, ask to be shown what would happen if you did heal from this now.

Once you have started on this journey, you may well be able to identify any other areas that still need to be healed in order to obtain your ideal body composition. Just add them to the list and continue on your journey.

This is the starting point to changing your life!

MEDITATION TO CREATOR OF ALL THAT IS

I want you to take a deep breath in and relax . . .
That's it . . . just relax . . . breathing deeper and relaxing more . . .

Allowing all the muscles in your body to relax . . . and as you relax more you imagine your feet firmly on the floor . . . and as your imagination drifts . . . as your feet firmly ground you to the floor . . . further down . . . through to the roots . . . further down and relaxing more with every breath you take . . .

You imagine yourself going further still . . . while safe in this space . . . . Your awareness goes even further . . . . And you relax even more . . . . And as you go further, you see that beautiful crystal in the middle of the earth . . . you can touch this beautiful crystal with your feet . . . grounding you safely to the earth . . . .

And now, still connected safely to the earth, your awareness comes back up through your body . . . up through your legs . . . relaxing your muscles in your feet . . . . Up through your legs . . . through all your muscles . . . relaxing more . . . as the energy comes up your body . . . . It strengthens . . . more energy . . . moving up . . . .

Your awareness now rises up through your body . . . . More and more energy gathers . . . coming up through your body relaxing you more and more . . . as your energy gathers your awareness comes up to the top of your head . . . . And you find yourself in your own beautiful bubble of light . . . protected and safe . . . .

And in your bubble of light you go up . . . up and up . . . past the stars and planets . . . and up even further . . . . Through dark light . . . and light . . . . Through dark light . . . and light . . . you may see ancestors . . . you may even ask them to help you . . . . Or you may just go past . . . . Up closer and closer . . . and now I want you to imagine that you are now in a jelly like substance . . . . And your bubble bursts . . . and you are safe . . . and free . . . and you find yourself swimming further up . . . . Up and up . . .

And then you see this beautiful iridescent white light. .and you go closer and closer until you are there . . . . In this beautiful iridescent white light . . . there with 'all that is' 'Creator of All That Is' and you are part of all that is . . . the warmth flows through every cell of your body . . .

And you make the command . . . .

> **"It is commanded that I have the strength and commitment to achieve my perfect bodyweight and perfect health, thank you . . . it is done . . . it is done . . . it is done . . . please show me"** . . .

Now watch . . . watch as you see yourself at that perfect bodyweight for you . . . imagine how that looks, how that feels to be at that perfect health . . . . And enjoy those feelings of what you can have in your life now . . . feel the strength . . . the commitment . . . the courage and determination you have . . . feel yourself now at that perfect weight . . .

And let us ask . . .

> **"It is commanded that I receive a physical healing for any past traumas to my body, for my highest and best good at this time . . . it is done . . . it is done . . . it is done . . . please show me"** . . .

Now watch . . . watch as you see yourself at that perfect bodyweight for you . . . imagine how that looks, how that feels . . . .

And let us ask . . .

> **"It is commanded that I receive an emotional healing for any past traumas to my body, for my highest and best good at this time . . . it is done . . . it is done . . . it is done . . . please show me" . . .**

Now watch . . . imagine how that looks, how that feels . . . .

And would you like to identify any of those habit's that get in the way? In the way of you having all you desire in your life . . . . . . think of them now . . . think of all the annoying habit's . . . that no longer serve your highest purpose . . . would you like to ask Creator of All That Is' . . . to free you from these habits . . .

> **"it is commanded that I free myself from these habit's . . . . Allowing myself to achieve my goals and desires . . . . Thank you . . . it is done, it is done, it is done . . . please show me" . . .**

And watch . . . imagine how that feels, how that looks . . . and feel yourself free and now at that ideal weight for you

Now I want you to imagine what you want in your life . . . . . . what you would ask for now . . . if you are part of all that is . . . this is what you would create in your life . . . imagine everything you want, everything that needs to be done at this moment . . .

I want you to see it done in your life . . .

I want you to say to yourself

"'Creator of All That Is' . . . this is in my life now . . . thank you . . . it is done . . . it is done . . . it is done . . . and so it Is" . . .

Imagine that it is in your life completely . . . imagine how it looks . . . . how it feels . . . . Enjoy those feelings . . .

You are taking away some beautiful tools and healings to create the life and body you wish to create . . . bring them all into your life now . . . feel the energy of unconditional love and healings . . . . .

Then take a deep breath in . . . you're still part of that white iridescent light . . . connected . . . knowing that you are part of 'all that is' and you can connect to 'Creator of All That Is' at any time.

You can have anything you wish to manifest . . . you know how to manifest all your desires . . . it can be in your life . . . and all these healings are part of your life now . . . as you integrate all these healings with grace and ease . . . and to keep with you throughout this lifetime . . . . .

Take another deep breath . . . . relaxing . . . knowing . . . and allow yourself a moment to enjoy these feelings . . . that's it . . . and now I want you to bring your awareness back to your body . . . .
Back to your feet grounding you to the earth . . . you feel your body . . . . You feel the chair . . . you are back in your space . . . your feet are back on the ground . . . and you are safe . . . and come back in your own time.

OTHER DOWNLOADS YOU MAY WISH TO TEST

I am fulfilled
I can achieve
I get healthier everyday
I am calm and collected
I am at my perfect weight
I live without fear of failing
I am worthy of all the good in life
I know when I am full
I am strong
I enjoy daily exercise
I know it's possible to eat right
My stomach is shrinking
I feel good about myself
The mirror is my friend
I am important
I avoid fatty foods
I take responsibility for what I eat
I eat slowly
I am calm and collected
I am my ideal weight for me
I enjoy good protein foods
I like fruits
Smaller portions of food are satisfying
Less bread is better
I like vegetables
I do eat right
I'm confident about releasing weight
I'm patient with myself

Every bite I eat is full of love
I become contented easily
I am supported
I am growing stronger
I am inspired to achieve
I know how to recognise when I am satisfied
I know the exercise that is for my highest good

I know what it feels like to live without
Feeling foolish
Feeling alone
Feeling out of control
Feeling I am wrong
Being a bother
People laughing at me
Feeling horrible
Being addicted to food
Being on the outside
Trying to please others
Rescuing others
Forcing my body
Without Scarcity`
Others betraying me
Feeling ugly
Needing to protect others
Feeling different
Being in the way
Feeling Strange
Being a freak
Being Useless
Feeling stupid
Feeling lazy
Being miserable
Feeling damaged
Hating myself
Torturing myself

Depriving myself
Without Scarcity
Abusing myself
Craving the wrong food
Ignoring my body
Harming my body
Fighting my body
Depriving my body
Cravings taking over my life
Being obsessed with food
Food dealing with my emotions
Food being an escape
Creating Fear
Being overwhelmed
Feeling left out
Feeling depressed
Creating depression
Feeling hurt
Being ignored
Being taken for granted
Having the world on my shoulders
Struggle
Being a victim
Feeling alone
Punishment
Being a doormat
Being Controlled
Suffering
Feeling deprived
Being separated from what I love
Being punished
People laughing at me
Having toxicity in my body
Being discouraged by my weight

HOW TO SET A "MACRO"

MACRO—This is what I agree with 'Creator of All That Is' when I ask for the healings

> - Read the Macro statement below
> - Decide on the Macro word you wish to use 'Teach it, fix it, heal it'
> - Go to 'Creator of All That Is' and state 'when I say 'teach it' it means all what I have just read out
> - You have now created your first Macro
> - Then Create a Macro using the 'live without' command using the same process

Macro statement

Have God's perspective, understanding, and definition of it
Your perspective, understanding and definition is the same
—It's possible and permissible for you
- You have the right to have/be/do/live it
- You know what it feels like to already have/be/do/live it
- You know when to have/be/do/live it
- You know that you're worthy and deserving to have/be/do/live it
- You know how to live your life on a daily basis having/being/doing /living it
- You do live your life on a daily basis having/being/doing/living it
- You know that it's safe to have/be/do/live it
- You know that only good will happen if you have/be/do/live it

You have all the power, tools and resources needed and know how to use them to have/be/do/live it, and you remember to do so

All above and how to **live without** a particular feeling:
  —without feeling it
  —without fear of it
  —without having to
  —without wanting to
  —without needing to

To replace a belief with whatever 'Creator of All That Is' chooses for my highest and best good at this time

And you receive all the downloads:
  —with grace and ease
  —in all languages
  —on all levels, and across all lifetimes
  —in the highest and best way
  —in all aspects, all angles and all areas of your life